# HOW TO Be a Resident Doctor Guide to Being Happy During Residency

# Table of Content

Introduction ................................................................................4
   How this book can help you ..................................................4
   How I got started on my journey ............................................6

HOW TO Manage Time ..................................................................10
   How to have a life outside of residency.................................10
   How to NOT get burned out during residency .....................20
   How to manage time when you are very busy.....................27
   How to find time to exercise..................................................33
   How to find time to do "extra" ...............................................37
   How to make time for your babies/kids................................39

HOW TO Work with Others ..........................................................44
   How to work with the nurses ................................................44
   How to work with attendings..................................................46
   How to work with peer residents...........................................50
   How to work with administration ............................................53
   How to NOT be the resident that no one likes.....................57

HOW TO do Your Work ................................................................64
   How to be organized..............................................................64
   How to take care of patients .................................................66
   How to present to attendings ................................................73
   How to write notes.................................................................75
   How to be a great doctor.......................................................78

HOW TO Do the Rest ...................................................................84
   How to study for board exam ................................................84
   How to get a job....................................................................87

How to determine what a job entails ..................................................... 89
How to determine where you want to work .............................................. 94
How to pay off your debt ........................................................................ 99
Final Thoughts ............................................................................................. 104
Thank you .................................................................................................... 106
About the author ......................................................................................... 107

# Introduction

**How this book can help you**

Everywhere you look, you can easily get information on how to BECOME a doctor – high GPA, pre-med courses, MCAT, board exams, applications, interviews, impressive resume, and so on. Rarely do you find a resource for HOW TO BE a doctor after you get "M.D." next to your name.

Often the expectation of residency is that you will bury yourself in work with no time for anything else. Common expectations for residents are that they will be miserable, exhausted, sleep-deprived, burned out, and even clinically depressed. No wonder nobody says, "I love my residency years." More often you hear residents say, "I hate my life" and "God, I can't wait 'til it's over!"

Most consider residency years as the hell you have to walk through to get to your final destination. I have seen many residents make poor decisions, breakdown in tears, live like dead zombies, get burned out, and placed on probation, all because, in my opinion, they did not know HOW TO be a resident.

How is it that there are how-to books and resources for everything under the sun, but not for how to be a resident doctor? My thought is that resident doctors often do not challenge the common misunderstanding that residency sucks. They put up with working long hours and struggling through their day because history and culture dictate that these grueling experiences are inseparable from being a resident. It's no accident that there are increased depression and suicide rate among residents.

The reality is that your experience of HOW your life will be is dependent on your answer to this question: What kind of residency life do I want? Do you want to be like everyone else in residency – overworked and burned out? Or, do you want to work fewer hours so you can spend quality time with your family or do whatever else is important to you? This book is about sharing with you how I achieved the happy, fulfilling life that I pursued during residency, so you can utilize similar tools to achieve yours as well.

You may wonder how I am the expert in this area. I'm not. However, I have always been passionate about teaching, living efficiently, and finding ways to make life better and easier to pursue greater quality of life. My hope is that this book will open your mind to find your ways to have what you want to get out of your residency by making mindful choices, thinking outside the box, and considering walking the road less traveled.

"Two roads diverged in a wood, and I –

I took the one less traveled by,

And that has made all the difference."

-Robert Frost-

## How I got started on my journey

When I started residency, I noticed that almost all residents were feeling burned out, unhappy, and miserable. Soon, I was feeling those emotions as well. I felt as though a dark cloud was hanging over me every day, every second of my life. I used to love making jokes and laughing, but it felt as though that happy part of my brain was turned off. I wasn't me.

Thankfully, I had a dawning moment when I met Dr. Grumpy (fake name) and Dr. Gray. When I was an intern working in a medicine rotation, I worked with several senior residents as part of a team. Usually there is one senior resident per team of interns and medical students. The senior resident manages the team, and also teaches, guides, and helps the team members when needed.

One senior resident, Dr. Grumpy, did not teach or help the team. She kept herself busy doing work that was not important. Yet, she always complained about how overworked she was and how she stayed so late working the night before. She was busy only because she created work for herself that was completely unnecessary.

On one occasion I had told her that I ordered 100cc/hr of saline water for a patient and she said I should change it to 110cc/hr without providing any reason. The 10cc/hr made no real difference, but she insisted and so I had to go down the stairs, look for the chart, change the order, tell the busy nurse, who then had to walk over to the patient and change the rate of flow. This was total waste of time for many people involved. This is an example of how Dr. Grumpy filled her day by being unproductive and creating work that didn't matter.

Also, Dr. Grumpy always had an "I-hate-my-life" attitude, complained all the time, and never smiled. You would think that this is the kind of person she had always been, but she wasn't. She was actually a really good friend of mine since before medical school. Because I took a year off during medical school, she graduated a year ahead of me and we lost touch. I remembered her as smart, funny, and just really cool to hang out with. I was initially excited to have her as my senior resident until I realized how much she had changed since she started residency. She wasn't fun or full of life anymore. Rather, she was mostly grumpy and looked miserable. All her complaining and negative attitude took a toll on me as well. I wondered if residency would also change me by the time I become a senior resident.

Fortunately, after two miserable weeks of working with Dr. Grumpy, she was replaced by Dr. Gray. Haaaallelujah! Thank God! Dr. Gray was truly like an angel, a gift from God. She always smiled, never complained, was appreciative, was very helpful, and even bought me pastries from Starbucks. She had a baby at home, so she told her team members that she would be pumping breast milk a few times during our shift, so we may end up seeing a boob or two. She would look at lab results, read notes, discuss patients, all WHILE pumping breast milk at the same time! So impressive! She utilized her time very efficiently and so we all left work at a reasonable time every day. However, what was most notable about Dr. Gray, unlike most other residents, was that she always looked happy.

I was so taken aback by the marked difference between the two senior residents doing the same job in the same environment. I realized I could choose to be like Dr. Gray or Dr. Grumpy, that I could CHOOSE to have a great residency experience, not the hell that I thought I had to walk through! I decided then to strive to be like Dr. Gray—efficient, productive, helpful, and most importantly, happy.

# HOW TO Manage Time

Managing your time well, at work and at home, is essential to doing more in less time and sparing yourself from burning out, so you can have more time to do what you want to do outside of residency.

## How to have a life outside of residency

During residency, finding free time does not just happen. You have to MAKE the time by living minimally and always thinking, "How can I do this quicker? How can I be more efficient?" Then your brain will notice and eliminate wasteful times. You are essentially squeezing what most residents do in 12 hours into 6-8 hours, so you are not necessarily working less, but working more in less time. The fewer hours you work, the earlier you can leave, and the more hours you have to play or do whatever you want to do outside of residency.

**Eliminate wasted time.** Most residents do not even notice that there are many pockets of wasted times during the day because they are not looking for them. Their mentality is "I'll leave when I can leave," allowing their environment to dictate their life. However, if you change your thinking and say, "I'm going to leave by 5 pm or earlier, no matter what," then YOU are the one who dictates your life. Then, you will notice that everything you do is done quickly and efficiently, and your brain will constantly look for solutions to eliminate wasted time.

When you work in a rotation, each day's schedule is about the same. In the first few days of a rotation, you will get a feel for how the day runs and will notice where time is consistently wasted. Then, you can figure out how to eliminate that wasted time or to fill it with something productive.

I worked with an attending who preferred to type her notes on a laptop that she carried after seeing each patient while the rest of the team, residents and medical students, waited for her to finish her notes. Though most attendings wrote their notes in their office after seeing all the patients with the team, this particular attending preferred that we all wait for her. What's worse is that she never learned to type properly, so she typed with two index fingers. We tried to make phone calls and get some work done while she was typing away with her two fingers, but we still could not do much.

What would you do in this situation? Would you just throw your hands up and say, "Oh well. I got unlucky with this attending. I guess I'll be working late for this rotation"? No! Do not accept any excuse to work late. It's easy to think, "Well, I can't tell her to learn to type. I can't tell her to do her notes in her office." If you are determined to meet your deadline of leaving by 5 pm, your brain will fill with solutions of what you CAN do, not with all the excuses of what you can't do.

What was our solution? We, the residents, offered to type for her and she happily agreed. This sped up our morning and we were done seeing all the patients HOURS earlier than we used to.

**Live with fewer distractions.** In life there is a lot of noise, which is anything that takes up your time that is unnecessary and distracts you from your path to meeting your goal. Eliminating noise means no Facebook, no shopping for clothes, no reading any non-required books, no new friends, no hobbies, no extracurricular activities, no latest electronics, and no unnecessary stuff. I know I sound like a drill sergeant, and realistically, you may not want to take away all these things. Maybe reading funny books at the end of the day is what you consider as part of being happy during residency. Maybe surfing on weekends brings you so much joy and helps you relieve stress that it becomes a must for you. Just know what your goal is, continue doing what makes you happy, and minimize everything else that does not meet that goal or brings you joy.

**Live with fewer possessions.** The more possessions you have, the more time is wasted buying and managing your stuff. For example, let's say you want to buy a TV for your apartment. It takes time to research the kind of TV you want, the size, features, brand, etc. You also need to buy a TV stand for your TV, so you do more research to find a compatible stand for your TV and the style of stand you like. Once you get the TV, you have to read the instruction, set up the TV, program the remote controls, and learn how to use all the functions. And what if your TV has a problem? You have to spend more time to call technical support and fix it or return it and get a replacement.

In addition, when you accumulate more possessions, you may outgrow your small apartment that's close to your work and have to move to a bigger space that is farther away. Then, you have added additional commute time to your day, all because you have too much stuff.

We live in a world where bigger and more are better, but NOT in the world of residency where smaller and less are much better.

**Live a minimal, simple life.** During residency, I had a friend who was complaining that she had to get up so early at 6:30 am to get to work by 8 am, though she lived close to work. I can guess why. Whenever I see her, she has full makeup on, nails always polished, nice outfits with matching jewelry, and hair perfectly done in many different styles. Just by looking at her, I can tell it would have taken a good chunk of her morning time to get ready.

I was once her as well, but during residency, my time to get ready in the morning was at most seven minutes. I moved quickly like on auto-pilot. As soon as I woke up, I brushed my teeth, splashed some water on my face, put on minimal make up, brushed my hair and pulled it back in a ponytail, wore my clothes, and then went out the door. Yes, all in seven minutes. How? Minimal, simple living.

Everyone asks the same question every morning: "Hm ... what should I wear today?" You look through some shirts thinking, "When was the last time I wore this? Hm... I wonder if this will look good with this." You may even pull out a shirt to wear and then change your mind and look for another one, something that you "feel like" wearing more than another. Whatever it is, people take time thinking about what to wear. The more clothes you have, the more decisions you have to make to say yes or no to a shirt or pants to wear for the day. You have even more decisions when you have a lot of shoes, jewelry, or accessories to choose from. As a resident, less is better.

During residency, my work attire consisted of three pants (black, dark gray, and light gray), one pair of black shoes, and about six shirts. Picking one pair of pants out of three is so much faster than flipping through ten or fifteen pairs of pants to decide what to wear. Wearing the same shoes means no time needed to make a decision on what shoes to wear. My hairstyle was always the same every day, pulled back in a ponytail, so I never had to decide how to do my hair. I didn't get my nails done, so no need to think about a matching outfit. I didn't wear jewelry then, so didn't need time to decide which jewelry to wear or to spend time putting it on. Having fewer decisions to make means faster speed.

Having a variety of nice clothes and shoes is important for some people, make them feel good, and is not something they want to change. Everyone has different preference. I have never been into fashion nor have I ever had much fashion sense, so saving time in this area of my daily routine was an obvious and easy one for me.

**What in your daily routine can you change to save time?** I know you may not want to hear this, but how about eliminating coffee? Many people are addicted to caffeine, which is the most addictive legal substance. I hear again and again, "I have to have my coffee to wake up." The culture also dictates that coffee is needed. I often see doctors in their white coats waiting in long lines at Starbucks in the morning. I had a friend who drove 15 minutes out of the way every morning (30 minutes round trip) to get Dunkin Donut coffee. If you quit drinking coffee, that is one less thing for you to spend time in the morning.

You may say, "I still have to have my coffee." That's fine. I just want you to consider the option of life of FREEdom, not having to depend on a chemical agent to get through the day, the "road less traveled" indeed. Imagine what more you can do with the money and time that you spend every day to get your coffee. And if you cannot give up your coffee, then maybe you can think of ways to shorten the time to get your coffee.

**Find comfortable shoes**. I wore one pair of black sneakers for most of my residency years. Before I wore sneakers, I used to wear nice dress shoes. However, there was a point where my back was hurting, so I started wearing black sneakers instead. I noticed I walked a lot faster wearing sneakers than dress shoes. Because I walked faster, I was zooming through the hospital, getting more stuff done in less time. So, I just continued wearing them even when my back no longer hurt. Honestly, I don't think anyone noticed or even cared. If they did, so what? Is someone going to charge me for not having style? I'm guilty as charged.

**Save time on cooking and eating.** Cooking a meal can take five minutes or more than thirty minutes. Eating a meal can also take five minutes or longer, especially if you are eating with friends. So, when you cook and eat, it can take ten minutes or over an hour. The point is to notice the time you take to cook and eat because this is another opportunity to save time.

When I cook, I cook in bulk so I can freeze or save some in the refrigerator to eat multiple times later on. I often cook a pot of soup or a large meal on a Sunday evening to eat left overs for a few days afterwards.

On most days at work, I eat and work at the same time. However, many residents eat and socialize. Sometimes when I pass the cafeteria, I see many residents in their white coats or scrubs, taking their time eating and talking. Don't get me wrong. I'm not trying to say, "Shame on you for eating and enjoying your conversations with your peers." I do want you to digest your food, and sometimes you do need to take a lunch break and socialize. However, if you take 30 minutes to eat lunch and socialize every day, the time just adds up.

**Strive to be efficient**. I was efficient at work and at home during residency, and I still strive to be efficient now. When I move around the house, I either run or walk fast. When I go grocery shopping, I know exactly what to buy, so I'm in and out very quickly. I don't go aisle to aisle pondering, "Should I buy this or that?" Whatever I do, cutting vegetables, folding laundry, putting kids' toys away, getting mail, I do them quickly. I gave up on neatness and perfection a long time ago.

You may ask, "So you move fast at work and at home. Wouldn't you be so tired?" No, because I have plenty of time when I turn my speed down to super slow. When I'm with my family, I take my time and mindfully enjoy every moment I have with them because they bring me so much joy and laughter. The other day during dinner, my four-year-old son picked up two green peas, put them together with his small fingers, looked up at me with big eyes, as though he had discovered something amazing, and excitedly said, "Mom! Look! If you put these together, you can make a small butt!" I laughed, and I have never seen green peas the same way since.

You may be filled with joy by spending time with your dog or fishing. That is the time to slow down and enjoy life. Life is about purposefully spending more time being happy and less time doing everything else.

**Learn from others.** When you wear the lens to be efficient, you will easily notice the areas in your life where you can be more efficient. You will also notice those residents around you who are even more efficient than you, so try to learn from them.

As an intern, I took 20-30 minutes to dictate an initial evaluation. I thought I was doing pretty good job on the time, but one day I saw my co-intern dictate in five to ten minutes! She spoke really fast with confidence. I thought I had to say "period" after each spoken sentence, but she didn't do that. I paused my dictation several times to gather my thoughts but she didn't do that. So, I learned how to dictate faster by watching her, and soon got my dictation down to five to ten minutes as well.

## How to NOT get burned out during residency

I used to think that getting burned out and working long hours are inevitable as a resident doctor. In the beginning of my residency, my life was just that. I felt like I worked all the time with barely any time with my family. I questioned, "Do I really have to put up with this for four years?" Many residents would say "yes," but even more would not even think to ask the question. Historically, working long hours and getting burned out are thought to be the typical experience of residency years, so residents just accept it and burn themselves out. Oh no. Not me! I'm no maverick, but I wasn't going to accept that. I loved my family too much to accept it, so I said, "I'm going to have great four years of my life during residency, creating many beautiful memories with my family!" And I made it happen.

It is amazing how easily you can achieve your goal when you are determined to make it happen. There is no secret. Everyone has achieved something that they felt that they MUST do, and it's just applying the same mind set.

When I was a resident, one of my resident friends confided in me how burned out she was and I truly felt badly for her. She looked like she was going to have a mental breakdown. I listened and provided emotional support because I knew that was what she needed the most at that time, but what I really wanted to say was to give her the same advices as below:

**Set yourself a goal, then you will figure out how to get there.** Once you set a goal and make it a MUST that you meet that goal, then it will happen. For example, if you set a goal to leave by 5 pm, then every decision you make during your day will help you reach that goal. You cannot think, "I wish we could finish early today" or "I hope I don't stay late again." When you wish and hope, you are like a passive observer, allowing things to happen to you. However, if you make your goal a MUST, then you play an active role in achieving that goal. Every decision you make, conscious and subconscious, you are thinking, "Will doing this help me to leave by 5 pm?"

In the beginning of my intern year, I was assigned to an attending, Dr. S, who tends to, let's say, not notice the time. I could only leave when she was done since we worked as a team, and she would often finish around 6 – 7 pm, sometimes 8 pm. I noticed my peer intern's attending finishing by 3 pm every day, so I knew that it wasn't the amount of work that was delaying my attending from finishing her work earlier.

After about a week, I figured out where Dr. S wasted most of her time and what I had to do to leave by 5 pm. Her main problem was that she chats a lot with ME! I admit she has very interesting and funny stories, but I still would rather come home early to see my kids. So, subtly, whenever she started chatting about non-patient related things, I would redirect her or sometimes kindly cut her off. You don't want to look like you are not interested in what your attending has to say and you don't want to be rude, so I just kept scooting her over to productivity. I would help her keep track of her time by saying, "Dr. S, we have to do __ and __ now," or "We have two more patients to see and we'll be done!" etc. I don't think she even noticed because I recall one time she said, "Wow, it's 5 pm. We're done already." That was because I set the goal to finish by 5 pm every day. I was determined to find the way and made it happen.

**Stop working and go home!** Sometimes even if you CAN leave on time, many residents don't, which blows my mind. They are just asking to get burned out. There will always be more work. You will never be completely done with work. So leave when you can and leave the rest of the work for tomorrow.

If you don't have family to go home to, you may think, "Well, I don't have anything to do tonight anyways, I'll just stay longer to finish doing this." If you think this way, you're the one who works 80 hours a week and complains how burned out you are and I'm the one who works 50 hours a week and has fun with my family the rest of the time. Would you rather work 80 hours a week or 50 hours a week? You're working almost twice as much and getting paid almost half as much per hour! Even if you have nothing to do at home, find something – read, watch TV, go to the gym, go shopping, cook a healthy meal – and take a mental break from work.

You may think, "Oh well, at least the patients are better cared for." No, that's not true. Working longer hours does not necessary mean you "cared" more or you provided more service to your patients. It may mean you are inefficient and stuck in the mentality that residents are supposed to work long hours.

**Get comfortable saying "No."** It's human nature to want to please others, and many people agree or say "yes" when they really should disagree and say "no" instead. If you haven't gotten comfortable with saying "no" in the past, you had better get there by the time you are a resident.

As a resident, many people—attendings, social workers, medical students, nurses, and patients—will ask you to do something for them, and for the most part, you actually have to do them, but NOT ALL. In fact, if you do everything that is asked of you, you will likely work long, late hours.

I remember a case manager who approached a resident around 6 pm, after that resident signed out and was about to leave. The case manager asked her to talk to a family member of one of the patients. The resident initially said no and said she'll call the following day, but the case manager pleaded with the resident, saying it would likely be a short conversation. As I was listening to this conversation next to me, I was internally rooting for this resident to stick to her guns and say "NO!" but the resident reluctantly agreed. The short conversation turned out to be over 30 minutes, time that this resident could have spent with her three-year-old daughter waiting for her at home.

I'm sure the family and case manager appreciated the resident for her time, but by saying "no," you are saying, "I'm important, too, and it's important for me to see my daughter before she goes to sleep." Work never stops and there will always be reasons why you should work more hours or stay late, but let the reasons why you should NOT work more and go home be stronger.

**Stop socializing.** Many people do not see socializing as waste of time, and rightfully so, because we are social beings and socializing is part of being human. However, some residents socialize too much and they don't even think about how much time they waste talking instead of working. So often the chatterbox residents work the latest, get burned out the fastest, and wonder why. They talk too much. Cut the conversation.

You may think, "But, you can't just cut people off when they are talking to you." Why not? I do it all the time. I fidget and turn my body to signal that I have to leave. If they don't pick up on that, I say something like, "Alrighty then, I gotta go."

You may think, "Oh, I can't do that. That's so rude." Who's being rude is all in perception. I think it's rude to prevent a person from working, so you can talk on and on about whatever is on your mind. Let's say that the person does think you are rude to walk away from the conversation. That may be a good thing. Hopefully, in the future, that person will find someone else to talk to instead of you.

**Be okay to NOT be a superstar**. By the time you are a resident, you have been the superstar of your high school, college, medical school, and probably all your extracurricular activities. You have all the awards and medals to prove what a superstar you are. That's your past and you need to keep that superstar in your past. As a resident, you don't have to be a superstar anymore because the price of superstardom is often getting burned out.

"Signout" is when a resident on call comes into work to take over your patients for the night until the following morning. After signout, you are relieved of your duty from your patients and you can go home, unless you CHOOSE to stay after signout to do more work, even though you don't have to! I remember one resident who stayed to work past 8 pm every day when the signout was at 5 pm. She had notecards for every patient, an organized binder, and all kinds of stuff—a classic work of a superstar. When I saw her working late every day, I told myself, "Oh no. Not me!"

When it was my turn to take over her position in the same site, I didn't make any notecards or color-coded binders. I worked very hard and efficiently, and EVERY DAY, I left as soon as the signout was over. No one would think of me as "one of the best residents ever," but I'm okay with that. The rewards for NOT being a superstar resident are saving myself from getting burned out and spending quality time with my kids before they go to sleep.

## How to manage time when you are very busy

Being busy is part of being a resident and it's not the kind of busy that most people think of. It is busy on steroids. There will be times where you have multiple urgent matters coming at you at the same time, demanding your immediate action. You either rise stronger or fall miserably. To rise, you have to be aware of how you are spending your time, prioritize your work, take care of your basic needs, do the bare minimal, and communicate.

**Be mindful of how you spend your time**. If you were to think about how you spent your day, or even just the past hour, and if there was a transcript of every word that came out of your mouth during that time, how would it look? It's one or the other: productive or wasteful. The more productive you are, the more likely you will finish what you have to do in a short amount of time. Therefore, the busier you are, the more mindful you should be to increase productivity and decrease wasteful time.

**Prioritizing your work.** Let's say in a given day, a resident has to do 30 tasks. What typically happens is that the resident knocks down one task at a time, keeps working at the list to complete as many tasks as possible. However, the reality is that if you do all 30 tasks, you will likely be going home late at night. In a busy day, working efficiently and eliminating wasteful time are important, but sometimes even that is not enough.

So then what do you do? You have to prioritize. Do the top 10 most important, most urgent tasks that you must do, and then plan to do the rest, based on priority, after the more important tasks are complete. If less important tasks remain incomplete by the time of signout, push them off for the next day and go home.

You may say, "Then, I have even more work the next day." Yes. So the next day, you prioritize again. The tasks that were low priority yesterday may become higher priority today or may remain low priority again.

You may say, "If it's low again, what if I don't get to it again?" Then, maybe tomorrow or the following day.

If you do everything you want to do, you will never leave the hospital. After knocking off the tasks in order of priority, you will likely have some non-urgent matters that you didn't get to do. I often say, "I'm done for the day. Those will have to wait until tomorrow," yet there are many overachieving residents who just cannot wrap their mind around the idea of calling it done for the day when there are items remaining in their task lists.

**"Go pee. Go eat that granola bar."** The busiest time during residency was when I was an intern during ER rotation. One to two months of ER rotation is required for most, if not all, of the residency programs. I felt most stressed during this rotation because of the fast pace in an unfamiliar territory.

I felt like I had to move fast because patients were sick or in pain, and waiting for me to put in the orders and take care of them. Because I moved so fast, I was also discharging patients fast. As patients left, I had more open space to accept new patients, and I moved fast to see those new patients. I was too busy to notice what I was doing to myself.

In a 10-hour shift, I was on such an adrenaline rush that I didn't pee even though the bathroom was literally five steps away. I didn't eat even though I had a granola bar in my pocket. I don't think I even drank water, but I was probably too busy to notice that I was thirsty. By the time I was done with a shift, I was completely drained of any ounce of energy. It was the most stressful and exhaustive work that I have ever done. Even in between my shifts when I was supposed to rest, I was stressed just thinking about how stressed I would be for the next shift.

I tearfully complained to my husband how I don't even have time to pee or eat a granola bar. My loving husband advised me, "Go pee. Go eat that granola bar. So what if a patient waits five minutes for you to use the restroom and get something to eat. It's NOT that big deal." It was an epiphany moment! That's right! They can wait! I'm going to pee!! And eat my granola bar!!!

Since then, I slowed down my pace, took care of my basic needs, and my stress level came way down. I still worked hard, but not to the point of craziness like I did before. I even took care of my patients better because I wasn't running around like a maniac.

**Do the minimum.** Another time when I was really busy was while I was on call. In the hospital where I worked, the weekday call work hours were from 5 pm to 7:30 am. You come in at 5 pm to get the signout, work through the night until 7:30am when you give the signout back to the resident working during the day. During this time, the resident on call may be the only doctor in his specialty working in the hospital. This resident on call is responsible for seeing patients in ER, in his unit, and in the hospital that pertains to his specialty. Therefore, most call nights are very busy. Because every call is so busy, you have to work efficiently, prioritize, and do the MINIMUM.

The objective is doing what is minimally necessary to get through the night until the other doctors, nurses, and hospital staff can take care of the patients the following morning. Therefore, ask and obtain only the information that you need for that night or that will change the course of care.

For example, when a patient comes into ER saying he hears voices, I ask if the voices are telling him to do something, like kill himself or others. If the patient says no, then I may discharge him from the ER. If he says yes, then I'll probably admit him for his or others' safety. Answer to this one specific question will determine two different directions of care. Questions like this is what you need to ask at the minimum. Sometimes when you are very busy, minimum is all you can do.

**Communicate to those waiting for you.** When you are on call, sometimes you can be in a situation where you get requests to see five patients within the span of ten minutes. What do you do?

Be efficient, prioritize, do the minimum, and communicate. Inform the staff who are waiting for your evaluation that you have five patients to see, you will get to their patient as soon as you can, and that their patient will likely be seen around ___ time. Then, they will understand your situation and will not get upset about how late you are.

I often hear residents say, "I'll get to him as soon as I can." The person who hears you say that is thinking, "What does that mean? In 30 minutes? In an hour?" They will assume what they assume, and you'll get paged again an hour later, "When are you going to see this patient?" So tell them up front to be considerate of their needs, and also so they'll stop bothering you.

## How to find time to exercise

As a resident, I was overweight by 15-20 lbs., but I was okay with that. At that time, I thought that a healthy lifestyle required a lot of time. I told myself, "I don't have time," which turns out to be the number one reason why most people do not exercise. Even after residency when I was working 28 hours a week, I was still using the same excuse, "I'm too busy. I still don't have time," when in reality, I don't like to work out and I would rather use that time doing something else.

After enjoying a little too much chocolate and a little too much comfort food, I came face to face with my ever growing rolly belly hanging off my pants like a muffin top. I had to either go to a bigger size pants or lose the weight. I decided to go shopping....for healthier food, and I started to exercise. I made a goal to lose the weight and put my health higher in priority.

As with everything you put your mind to, I figured out how to make exercise work for me. My issue with exercise has been that I don't like to feel like I'm working out and I don't like to take up time in the day to exercise. So, I came up with two solutions that worked for me.

**First, I tie exercising to something fun or productive.** For example, I take Zumba classes on Friday mornings so I dance and have fun while getting a good exercise. I also go to the gym on Tuesday mornings, and I watch YouTube videos about different topics I'm interested in while I work out on the elliptical. The other day, I watched a video about Amazon Kindle publishing since I'm trying to figure out how I can publish this book. I got so into learning about it that 45 minutes passed in a blink of an eye. By the time I was done, I was breathing hard and sweating profusely.

Before I did this, I used to flip through TV channels while on the elliptical, watch some news, some reality shows, or whatever seemed interesting. However, I was never really into what I was watching, so I was aware that I was working out, trying to pass time, and frequently watching the clock to finish at the 30-minute mark. When I was watching YouTube on a topic in which I was really interested, I barely looked at the clock.

Sometimes I swim, and this is the time when I plan out my immediate goals like brainstorming the contents of a chapter of this book, strategizing my next project, and thinking about my long term life goals and what I want to accomplish. I keep my mind busy and productive, so I don't make space in my mind to "think" that I'm swimming to exercise.

**Second, I add mini-exercises throughout my day.** This is what I wish I had done as a resident because mini-exercises are perfect for busy people. To get on board with what mini-exercises are, you have to break your concept of what a typical exercise is.

When you think of exercise, you think what? Going to gym, aerobic classes, and going for a run. Whatever it is, most people think at least 30 minutes of working out. In actuality, in addition to 30 minutes exercise, you have to take time to get ready, walk/drive to where you plan to exercise, get back from the exercise, and take a shower afterwards, all of which can easily take over an hour.

As a resident, time is hard to come by. So many residents either don't exercise or do it once or twice a week on a day off. Instead of spending a chunk of my day to exercise, I break it into little pieces and spread them throughout my day, working them INTO my schedule.

There are many pockets of wasted time during your day that you can find to squeeze in some mini-exercises, like repetitions (reps) of lunges, squats, side leg lifts, push-ups, sit-ups, or other reps that targets various muscle groups. Here are some examples:

- When I put my food in the microwave for two minutes, I do some reps while I wait.
- When I'm waiting for the gas pump to fill my car, I'm doing my reps next to my car. You may ask, "Don't people look?" Yes. I smile and say, "Hello." I'm not trying to make a scene, just doing some lunges. I hope I motivate those lookers to do the same.
- When I'm in a conference room for a meeting, waiting for others to come, I'm doing my reps.
- When I'm waiting for the rest of my family to come to the door to leave the house, instead of yelling at them to hurry up, I use that time to do some reps.
- If I'm in my office and in between seeing my patients, I often do about five minutes of reps with the help of a chair in my office.

- When I'm putting my kids to sleep at night, I'm doing some sit-ups next to their bed.
- When I'm watching TV at night, I'm either stretching, doing sit-ups, or working on my arms with dumbbells.
- When I go grocery shopping, I run or walk very quickly to and from the store to the car and vice versa. I know some people watching me may think, "That girl really is in hurry to get her milk." I'm in hurry alright, but to get rid of my rolly belly.
- When my kids play in the playground, I use the bars, steps, or whatever I can find to help me do some reps while watching the kids.

The key is to do these mini-exercises routinely as a habit, so you don't even think that you are doing them. Now I do a lot of these reps automatically without much thought. So I always watch TV from the floor while doing some reps. I quickly go into lunges as soon as I press start on the microwave. I run/fast walk out of my car to a store without even telling myself that I should run/fast walk.

## How to find time to do "extra"

By the time you are a resident, you are plucked from the cream of the crop of the cream of the crop. To be a doctor, the competition is fierce. When I was accepted to medical school, the acceptance rate was about 1%. Getting into your preferred residency program is another intense competition. By the time you are a resident, you are one of a group of super smart, impressive, overachieving residents, who has always done extra to have impressive resume and applications. For many, this hunger to do extra remains, even as a resident.

However, the reality is that you are done! No more competition! No more need to be an overachiever. Even if you want to go into fellowship, it is not nearly as competitive as getting into medical school or residency. So, relax.

Do extra work ONLY if you want to. It is okay to just do what you are required to do. If you really want to do that extra something—research, write an article, serve on a committee, whatever you want—then the best time is the last couple of years of your residency when you have fewer calls and a more reasonable work schedule.

What I often noticed is residents feeling pressured to publish research, write articles, and volunteer for different programs on top of their demanding work week. If you enjoy doing them and you have time, then go for it! That could be your reason to be efficient and leave work early. But if you don't, then don't do it.

I had two small children while I was a resident, so every free time I had I wanted to spend with them. Sure, I was encouraged to do research, write articles, and be more involved in various activities, but I politely said I didn't want to do them. My residency director and the program staff were awesome in that though they encouraged, they neither pressured me nor made me feel guilty about not doing anything extra. During my fourth year (the last year of my residency) I had more free time since I didn't have any calls, so I volunteered to head the Teaching Committee and took on a few additional responsibilities, which I WANTED to do and I really enjoyed doing.

## How to make time for your babies/kids

The best time to have a baby is any time because there is no good time to have a baby. Having a baby requires so much time and money, so the decision as to when to have a baby should be a conscious, well-planned one. Most residents choose to have a baby later in their residency years because the work hours are easier at that time, but some choose to have early for their own reasons.

When I started residency, I had a two-year-old son, and my husband had a demanding career. When we were planning to have our second child, we decided to give birth between my first and second year of residency. I wanted a year off for my second son as I had with my first, to breastfeed and have a year of bonding with him. My residency program hires a second year transfer resident. So I asked to leave after my first year, so the residency program could hire two second year transfer residents when I began my leave, and, when I returned from leave, they wouldn't need to hire a transfer. With this schedule, my absence did not add any additional calls for my fellow residents and did not decrease the number of residents supporting the hospital.

However, most residents do what most residents do, which is to take about six to eight weeks of paid leave, and sometimes a little longer without pay. Then, they put their babies in someone else's care, pump breast milk every few hours if they choose to continue breastfeeding, on top of carrying all the responsibilities as residents. I, personally, did not want to take on so many responsibilities at home with a newborn and at work as a resident, but this is what most resident mothers do. Frankly, I have been quite impressed by how well they do it, but there are other options.

**Hire help**. Hiring a help should be seriously considered if you have kids and if you can find means to afford it. Many people do not think to hire help if they can do the work themselves, which works if you are not a resident and have a life with a lot of free time. When you are a resident, managing time well is essential to happy living. So, hiring help is like outsourcing the work you don't want to do, so you can have time to do what you want to do. It is like duplicating yourself, so that one self is cleaning while the other self is working or playing with the kids. It is also like gaining additional two to three hours to your 24-hour day. You are exchanging money for additional time you need in the day.

The most powerful tool I had to help me through the residency years, that gave me quality time to spend with my children, was my own mother. She lived 30 minutes away but chose to live with me Monday through Friday for a year while taking care of my one-year-old son. She also cooked and cleaned. Even after a year, she came over three times a week to help with picking up kids from daycare, cooking, and house work. My father helped as well. I could not have done so well during residency, as a mother and a doctor, if it weren't for my parents. I appreciated and paid them for their help, but the amount of work and care they provided was beyond what any hired professionals could have provided.

A fellow resident had her mother move from out of state and live with her during residency to take care of her young child. Another resident with two young children hired help for a few hours a day to clean and do laundry, which she said was very helpful. She found her help from Care.com, and she paid $15 per hour.

Imagine scenario 1. You come home from work. Kids are already picked up from daycare, fed by your hired help, and they are happy. Your food is ready on the table. You eat and play with your kids, while your help cleans the dishes and folds laundry.

Imagine scenario 2. You hurry to leave work so you can pick up the kids before the daycare closes. You rush through traffic, almost get into an accident, but just make it in time before you have to pay penalty for late pickup. When you pick up your kids, you notice they're the last two kids to be picked up. You do the walk of shame, leaving the daycare. Kids are already complaining how hungry they are on the drive home and they are cranky. You come home and it's a mess from early in the morning when you didn't have time to clean up and do the dishes. Your kids wait restlessly while you prepare their food. After you give them their food, you are stuffing yourself with whatever food you can eat. Then, the kids ask you to play, but right then, your husband comes home from work. Now you prepare food for him, all the while your kids are asking to play and help with their Lego set. You play for a little bit, but it's already time to get them ready for bed. After they go to bed, then you do the dishes, laundry, clean up, and finally pass out from exhaustion.


You choose.

# HOW TO Work with Others

As a medical student, you are on your own. You take your own exams, work on your own projects, and you do your own thing. As a resident, you have to work well with others because you mostly work in teams and rely on others. How well you do often depends on how well they do. Sometimes how stressed you are has more to do with the social relationships than the actual work.

## How to work with the nurses

**Listen and consider what your nurses have to say**. As a resident, and especially as an intern, the seasoned nurses have more practical experience than you have. In certain situations they would probably make better decisions than you. Knowing this, if I feel stuck and don't know what to do, I ask a nurse, "What would other doctors do in this situation?" This not only helps clarify the immediate decision, but it also builds trust and rapport with the nursing staff.

However, don't just assume your nurses know better because they do not have the kind of medical training you do. Utilize their knowledge, but always keep in mind that you are the doctor, the one who's ultimately responsible for your patient's care.

Also, if you make a decision or order something, and the nurses tell you it may not be a good idea, then listen to them and seriously reconsider your decision. Nurses generally just follow doctors' orders without questioning, but when they do question, you had better listen. Even if you think you are right, run it by another doctor, just to make sure.

I recall overhearing an intern's phone call with a nurse. The intern was yelling at the nurse saying, "Just do what I ordered!" I felt badly for that nurse for how that intern was speaking to her. Later I found out that this intern ordered a large dose of potassium for a patient. The nurse was trying to tell the intern that it was too much and the intern just yelled at her, telling her to do what she ordered.

Thankfully, the patient was okay and was given medication to help decrease the potassium level back to normal. However, the incident was reported to the senior resident, attending, and higher ups. This could have turned out really badly for that patient, who unfortunately had a doctor who wouldn't listen to her nurse.

**You want the nurses to like you**. I have learned early that your work life can be a lot better if you are on the nurses' good side. Nurses are the gatekeepers, your frontline army, your shield, and they look out for you. So, be kind and appreciative even when you are sleep-deprived and tired.

In one call night, I was so busy working through the night that I felt like I was becoming delirious from exhaustion. The word "tired" does not do justice to describe how incredibly drained I was that night, physically, mentally, and emotionally. I was finally done at 4 am and was able to lay down to rest. Surprisingly, I didn't get paged for next two hours and had the most restful two hours of sleep. Later when I went to the nursing station, I noticed a fax that was meant for me to review for a possible transfer patient. The nurse told me, "Yeah, that came in an hour ago, but I knew you had a rough night, so I wanted you to get some more sleep." I was so grateful and moved by her thoughtfulness that I almost had an ugly cry moment. Thankfully, I was able to compose myself. After all, I worked in the psychiatric unit. I didn't want look like I was losing my mind.

**How to work with attendings**

**Make your attending's life easier**. During a typical day, you have dozens of decisions to make – what antibiotics to order, what doses of pain medications to prescribe, what lab work to order, etc. Make all these decisions yourself. Do all the work and then ask for approval. Nothing makes an attending feel better than to know all the work is done, and he doesn't have to do anything.

What I often hear is a resident saying, "This patient is___. What should I do?" Think of what you should do first and present it, so that your attending knows that you are a thinking doctor, capable of making decisions, not just a secretary. Better to say something like this: "Dr. H, this patient is ___ with diagnosis of ___ and doing ___ and I'm thinking of treating with ___ because of ___." If Dr. H disagrees, he will let you know and you will learn from it. If Dr. H agrees, he will think you are smart and will appreciate that he didn't have to do anything.

When I was a senior resident, I was on call with an intern, Dr. N. She received a consult request to evaluate someone in ICU. Dr. N called me and said, "Well, I've never done this kind of consult before, so I don't know what to do." I said okay, and I taught her what to do. She is more of a typical resident with typical mentality of "I don't know. I'm just an intern. You teach me." So I did, and probably spent about 30-45 minutes.

Then, on another call, I was working with another intern, Dr. S. She got a call for consult as well and she also had never done this kind of consult before. She chose to see the patient first, did her evaluation, wrote up a note, and then called me to ask if she did okay. Her evaluation and note were great. I asked her how she did it since it was her first consult evaluation. She pulled out a small book from her pocket and said she used it to help her. I spent less than five minutes giving some feedback to make her note better.

Develop a habit of thinking for yourself and making decisions before you consult with more senior doctors. This will not only help you quickly become a more independent doctor, but you will be loved by your attendings as well.

**Be a good secretary to your attendings.** Keep your attendings organized and on schedule. Not every attending is efficient and good with timing, so sometimes you have to keep them on track, and remind them of meetings, supervision hours, etc. This is to your benefit because if they waste time chatting and doing non-work related stuff, then it's also your wasted time as well.

I like to keep things organized, set alarms for reminders, always have pen and paper plus other commonly used items. Some attendings work without anything in hand and go about the day without much focus or direction, creating multiple pockets of wasting time. So when I see that the attending needs a pen, I pull out my extra pen for him to use before he even asks. When he is done with one patient, I tell him the room number for the next patient to see, which is the nearest room so we don't have to waste time walking so far. When it's close to meeting time, I remind him that we have a few more minutes until we have to go to the meeting, so he can speed things along. Every little thing like these decreases wasted time and speeds up the day. Plus, who doesn't want to be catered to?

Attendings will appreciate how easy you have made their work life and, one way or another, they will also reciprocate and make your life easy as well. Sometimes they even let you go home early.

## How to work with peer residents

When I work with my peer residents I think about Matthew 7:12, "So in everything, do to others what you would have them do to you…"

**Give a good signout.** A good signout is when you know your patients' diagnosis and plan, and you say to the resident taking your patients, "There is nothing for you to do."

When I was an intern, on my first day of ER shift, I was clueless. It was fast pace work, which required quickly making multiple decisions. Somehow I barely got through my first shift, but I was so busy I didn't realize it was time for the next resident to take over the shift. When the resident came and asked for my signout, I gave her the list of patients I had. She asked what were their diagnosis, what was the plan, what had been done, what tests were ordered – it was as though I was in an interrogation room with a lit lightbulb dangling in front of me, beads of sweat coming down my forehead, and my only response was, "I don't know. I don't know!" I could see from her stiffened expression that she was upset. I apologized, but that didn't hold her back from letting me have it. She yelled, "This is the worst signout I ever got!" Ouch. I felt so bad that since then I tried my best to give the best signout ever!

Call signout is different from ER signout. Usually, the resident on call comes in around 5 pm and gets signout from the resident who had been working during the day. Bad signout is, "If you have time, can you do the physical exam, call the family, follow up on this lab, etc." If it can wait until the next morning, then don't ask the resident on call to do it over night. Being on call is super busy, so if the resident on call has time, he should be resting, not doing your work that could wait or that you didn't get to do. As mentioned above, what you should be saying is, "There is nothing for you to do." If you have to stay late to make this statement, you should.

You may say, "I'm not just going to stick around for a lab result...etc." You're right. Then, you should say something like this, "There is nothing for you to do NOW, but please follow up on ____. You should expect the results around ____. If the results say ____, please do____." Also, write these instructions down on the signout sheet as well, so the resident on call doesn't have to write it all down. Make it easy on the resident on call and only ask to follow up if someone must follow up that day. For example, you are looking for hemoglobin hematocrit level to see if the patient is bleeding internally or not. That's something that cannot wait until the following morning.

**Be nice and help each other**. As a resident, you often rely on other residents from different departments to help you with your patients. For example, if your patient has a heart disease that is more complicated than you or your attending can handle, then you call for a consult to cardiology resident. However, calling for any consult can be challenging.

In the hospital I worked, no one liked getting a call for a consult because that meant more work for the resident receiving the request. Sometimes you have to be like a salesperson on the phone, making a pitch to say why this is a legitimate consult request. The resident receiving the consult request often looks for any excuse to not see your patient and argues with you about why a consult is unnecessary. Sometimes the resident even refuses to see the patient, and often is mean about it, making you feel like an idiot. Calling for consult was one of those things I hated to do because after I hang up the phone, I felt emotionally bruised.

When it was my turn to receive a psychiatry consult request, I made sure that I always accepted a consult request and I was nice about it. I never argued, and I always thanked the resident for the consult, no matter how stupid it was.

I once got a psychiatry consult request and when I asked for the consult question, the resident on the other line said, "He just needs someone to talk to." Are... you... SERIOUS?! I'm a medical doctor, not "someone to talk to." Go find a family member or a friend! In fact, why can't YOU talk to him?! Urrr! I could have said any one of these, but I chose to say, "OK, I'll evaluate the patient to see if there is any psychiatric diagnosis and what we would recommend. Thank you for the consult. I'll talk you later with our recommendations."

## How to work with administration

Administration usually includes residency director, residency assistant director, chair of the department, chief resident, and residency coordinator. They are your angels who work tirelessly to help you get through your residency successfully and become a great doctor.

**Do not bother the administration**.  Before you ask the administration to do something, know that it will likely be a bigger battle, be more complicated, involve more people, and take much longer than you think.  So, seriously consider if it's worth the time and energy to bring it up to the administration because in most cases, it's not worth it.

When I was an intern, I noticed that I had five more work days than my peers because I happened to work in medicine rotation during winter holidays.  I thought, "not fair!"  So I went to the administration to ask for five additional days off from work "to be fair."  Well, it didn't happen and I was unhappy about it then.  However, looking back, I see that the administration made the right decision to not give me extra vacation days.  If I had gotten five additional vacation days, then the administration would have had to assign someone else to work in my place for those days.  Not only that, what about that one other intern, who also worked few more days than everyone else?  The administration would have had to give her additional vacation days too "to be fair."  As an intern, I didn't think of all these consequences of my asking for a few days off.  Now I think, "So what that I got five more days of work.  Life is not always fair."

**Do not make excuses to not work**. Residency work can be very challenging, so residents often look for REALLY good excuses to not work and expect the administrators to make changes to accommodate for their absences. However, one resident's absence can have ripple effect and disrupt many people's schedule, who won't be so happy about it. Also, what you consider to be a really good excuse may not be for others.

Dr. Gray had to pump breast milk at least three times during her work, but she didn't consider that as an excuse to not work. She worked while she pumped. I had a medical student who came in to do his call shift with me. He limped his way into the call room with crutches, a full leg cast, and bandages around his head and one of his arms. He looked like he just came back from war. One look at him and I was like, "What are YOU doing here?" He told me he was hit by a car while crossing the street the day before, but he was "okay." I told him that he could go home and rest. He said he didn't want to, that he would rather be on call and learn. This medical student and Dr. Gray chose not to make their situations into an excuse to avoid work.

**Work together**. If you do have an excuse and can't work, then you have to work WITH the administration to figure out a way to make up those times. I knew of a resident whose baby was very sick, so she was absent for a significant period of time to take care of her baby. When she came back to work, she had multiple meetings with the administration to find ways for her to get back on track. She eventually had to extend her residency by a year and make up all the missed calls. She even had to take calls in her last year of residency, which is not typical. The administration and she worked together to personalize her schedule, so she could make up all the work that she missed while she was away and meet all the requirements to graduate from residency. This did not necessarily mean that it was going to be fair or to her liking.

**Appreciate**. Residents often come to administration with complaints, but how many come to say thank you? Very few. Only in the last year of my residency when I had a chance to help the administration for a task, I realized how much work they put in to help the residents have a wonderful experience, how much they give without being noticed or appreciated, and how much effort they put in to be fair to every resident.

My residency director, Dr. Catapano, is one of the most generous and considerate people I know. She would often host parties for the residents in her home. She bought gifts for individual residents for various occasions. She even got Georgetown cupcakes, the BEST in the area, for all the residents during our residency retreats. She was like a loving mother figure to all of us, and I feel so blessed to have been part of a residency program that was led by her.

Being part of the administration is a tough, thankless job. The least we can do is to say, "Thank you."

## How to NOT be the resident that no one likes

**Don't make excuses.** Residents often make excuses. "I couldn't do a physical exam because…" "I was late because…." "I didn't do what you asked because…" "I need to take a week off because I'm mourning for the death of my cat" (a true story).

No one likes to hear excuses and frankly, there is no such thing as a "good" excuse. Every excuse is bad. Do not put yourself in a situation where you have to think about an excuse because you did not do something. Put reminders in your alarm clock. Come to work earlier. No more excuses. Why? After too many excuses, you will be considered unreliable and to have poor work ethics.

Once you graduate from residency, you will be in contact with other alumni of your program and have a network of professional relationships. Think about the impression you make on others when you are not meeting your responsibilities and always making excuses. I often get calls from residents from classes below me asking for job opportunities in the Northern Virginia area or at my workplace. If I know you as someone who is often late or makes excuses, how can I tell my colleagues or boss, who is considering to hire you, what a great resident you are?

One day you will wonder, "How come that attending partnered with Joe to do the research project and not me? How come I didn't get that opportunity? How come the residency director did not ask me to head the Committee?" "How come that senior resident didn't tell me about that clinical site and instead told Jane about it?" If you make too many excuses, people's impression of you is that you are unreliable, so who will give you responsibilities, opportunities, or even a job after residency?

**Do not complain.** Residency life is not easy, so often you hear residents complain about all kinds of stuff. I used to complain as well, but I realized that complaining serves no purpose, wastes time, and puts you and the person you're talking to in a foul mood.

So, do not complain and stay away from others who do. You may say, "But everyone I know complains. I can't avoid everyone." That's true, but I'm sure you can think of that one or two residents who complain almost all the time. You naturally empathize and contribute to their complaining, but what do you get out of it? You just feel lousy, upset, or depressed. When I see from a distance that I'm about to cross path with a resident who I know complains A LOT, I do a U-turn, pretend I'm talking on the phone, or hide behind a big guy and pretend I didn't see him. Do whatever it takes to avoid interacting with those who complain and drain your happy spirit.


Also, reflect and be mindful of your words as well. Every time you catch yourself complaining, step back and say, "Oh no. I'm not going to waste any energy on negativity." Instead speak encouraging, uplifting, and positive words. Ephesians 4:29: "Let no corrupting talk come out of your mouths, but only such as is good for building up as fits the occasion, that it may give grace to those who hear."


**Do not check your phone.** Many people are addicted to checking their phones. I see people checking their phones everywhere – in the middle of rounding, in a meeting, in classes, in patient rooms, in bathrooms, EVERYWHERE.

Next time you are in an auditorium full of attendings, residents, and staff, listening to a world-renowned guest speaker, look around you. You will see how many people have their heads down, looking at their cellphones. The speaker may not notice if one or two people are not paying attention and looking at their cellphones, but when more than half the audience is looking down at their phones, it would be hard to not notice.

Even in a small group setting, look around you. When I was teaching a group of three residents, one or two would inevitably be checking their phones. When someone is trying to communicate with you and you are checking your phone, you are basically saying, "I'm not listening. I don't care what you have to say. Checking my phone is more important than you."

**Be on time.** No one will remember if you are late one or two times. However, if you are consistently late many times, you will leave a lasting negative impression.

People talk. People notice. You may not think it's a big deal to be late, but others do. If you are late, you are basically saying, "I'm more important than you. My time is more important than your time. I shouldn't wait for you. You should wait for me. So I can be late." Being late implies that you do not manage time well and that you are inconsiderate, selfish, and disrespectful. Punctuality matters!

I knew of one resident who was always late to everything. I noticed he was supposed to come to signout at 5 pm to take over my patients, but I knew that he would be late, yet again. I was already upset knowing it was he who was coming for call duty because I can't leave unless he comes to take the signout. Another resident in the room also noticed his name for the day's call and expressed her sympathy, saying, "Yeah, he's always late. He's such a ___." An attending in the room overhearing us asked, "Who?" When we said the name, she said, "Yeah, he's always late with me as well," and she continued complaining about how irresponsible he is and how it's not right that he always makes others wait for him. It was obvious that this particular resident consistently being late bothered everyone, which instigated other negative comments about the resident. Being late might not have been a big deal to the resident, as he was always late, but it was obviously a big deal to others, which also opened the door to a flood of negative comments about him.

**Respond to emails.** You would think this is obvious, but surprisingly many interns and residents do not respond to emails. It may be that we are bombarded with so many emails every day that you end up just skimming through, thinking you'll respond later, and later you forget.

There are emails that you can just put aside and there are those to which you MUST reply. If the email is asking for a response, you must reply as soon as possible especially if the email is from your superior (e.g., administration, medical director, or attendings). If you don't respond, it builds frustration in the person who emailed you and is waiting for your response, and leaves a lasting negative impression of you.

You may say, "But I was waiting for____ before I could respond." Then, you should reply to the email right away saying, "I'm waiting for ____ and I'll get back to you as soon as I know, hopefully by the end of this week. If not, I'll let you know." Not responding to emails gives the impression that you are irresponsible or that you consider the email not important enough for you to respond. You DO NOT want your superiors to think that their emails are not important enough for you to respond!

**Emotion reflects emotion.** The emotion that you see is often the emotion that you feel. When you watch reality shows where real people show true sadness and tears, do you also notice tears forming in the corners of your eyes? When your sibling is angry and yelling at you, do you also find yourself responding with the same heated emotion? When you see your children happy and laughing, doesn't that also make you happy? Exhibiting a particular emotion draws out the same emotion in others.

As a resident, I hated being on call late at night because that's when many people were mean and irritable. They would hang up on me, yell at me, all kind of rudeness, that I would never get during the day. I wondered why. Looking back, I know I tended to get irritable and cranky when I was sleep-deprived and tired. Who knows if it was my irritability that caused others' irritability, or vice versa. It was probably a little bit of both.

Knowing what I know now, I consciously surround myself with happy, positive people because I want to stay in that kind of environment. You become whom you surround yourself with.

# HOW TO do Your Work

Taking care of patients, writing your notes, and presenting to your attendings take up a significant portion of your day as a resident, so doing these well, thoughtfully and efficiently with good organization, is essential to finishing work on time and going home early.

## How to be organized

The right amount of organization is very important to being efficient. Some residents spend too much time organizing, delaying doing the actual work. Many residents skip the initial organization to save time and jump right into doing the work but that approach can end up costing more time in the long run.

When you start your intern year or any rotation in a different hospital setting, the first challenge is getting to know the system. Every hospital has a different electronic medical system that's not always user friendly. Each rotation has its own procedures, contacts, and phone numbers for different services. Write them down in your phone or on a notepad that you will carry every day. So the next time you need that information, it's readily available to you. This saves you time in the future, so you do not have to look for that information that you had searched already.

I used to call "0" for the operator to get all the numbers including for Environmental Service, fourth floor nursing station, Information Technology, who is on call, etc., but it's faster if you write these numbers down and use your own notes because sometimes the operator is busy, gives a wrong number, gives several possible numbers, or doesn't know the number.

One time I needed to get the number for a surgery consult. The operator gave me a number, but in the end, I paged and spoke to three different doctors, one telling me to call the next, to finally figure out which number I was supposed to call. Because I wrote down the correct number at that time, I didn't have to page three doctors again the next time I needed a surgery consult.

Another organizational tool is a "to-do" list for the day with a checkbox in front of each task. Once you are done with a task, you put a check mark in the box. As a resident, you have many responsibilities that come up throughout the day. Do NOT rely on your memory to get them done because you will get distracted and forget. Having a list not only is a reminder but also keeps you productive because at any spare time, you have a list of things to do. At the end of the day when you see your long list with a bunch of check boxes, it makes you feel good to know how much you have accomplished.

## How to take care of patients

Taking good care of your patients is not all about how much you know. It is HOW you serve your patients that separates a caring doctor from the rest.

I often have patients come to me and complain about their previous doctors, who "didn't care," "only gave me prescriptions," "barely talked to me," and "didn't listen." I was probably one of those doctors as well, more concerned about the science of treating the patient's illness than the patient.

I recall shadowing one doctor who was very knowledgeable, kind, and friendly to his colleagues, but that caring person disappeared when he was with patients. He barely made eye contact, asked only a couple of questions, wrote the prescription, and sent them on their way. When patients tried to talk a little more, he immediately cut them off and again, scooted them out the door. One patient after another, he had the same demeanor, asked the same questions with same disconnect. There was no relationship. But maybe he just didn't want to have relationships with his patients. Being a doctor, after all, is just a job, or is it?

**Be the kind of doctor you want as a patient.** When you are a patient going to a doctor's appointment, you know almost immediately if that doctor really cares or if seeing you is just a job to him. It is in his smile, his eye contact, his patience in listening, and his attention to details. Well, now you are the doctor. Your patients will know, just like you did as a patient, whether you sincerely care or if they are just one of many patients you have to see in that day to do your job.

Is being a doctor just a job to you? And, if it is, then there's no shame in that since that's what most people think of their jobs. However, you have the privilege to be in both positions, as a doctor and a patient, so you can choose to be the kind of doctor that you would want to have as a patient.

**Make the patient feel special.** Prior to medical school, I worked at the Mayo Clinic and I had the chance to observe a doctor who had the most incredible rapport with his patients. I could tell that patients loved him and it was evident that he made every one of them feel important and special. He had a trick up his sleeve that I learned, which has been one of my most valuable tools that I use to connect with my patients.

With every patient that this doctor sees, he asks for or picks up something unique about that patient. Maybe it's that a patient loves to go hiking, or has a dog name Pepper, or has a daughter named Susie who's a cheerleader. The more specific and personal the better. He writes this personal information on the front page of the patient's chart, and each time that patient comes, he quickly glances at what he wrote and asks, "So, how's Pepper these days?" or "Did you go on any good hiking trails lately?" or "Is Susie still cheering away?"

The looks on the patients' faces were priceless! I could see their thoughts from their glowing faces with widened eyes, "No way! How could he remember that from months ago?" "He cared enough to remember," "He must be so smart to remember that," "He listened," etc. You can see how special the patients feel and how much they think of this doctor.

This is how you connect with your patients. This is how they think you are the greatest doctor in the world and trust you with their health. This is how your reputation spreads by word of mouth and soon you will see your patients' families and friends.

**Give patients the freedom to choose.** The best medication for the patient is not what's the best medication for the illness, but the best medication that the patient is willing to take.

Gone are the days when you go to a doctor's appointment and the patient does exactly what you tell him to do. Now patients have Google, support groups, Facebook, Wikipedia, and many resources from which they can obtain free medical information. So, a more current response to a given recommendation is, "Well, I googled it and it says\_\_\_\_," "I read online that \_\_\_\_, so I decided not to take the medication."

What I learned about human thoughts and behavior as a psychiatrist is that no one likes being told what to do. In fact, when you tell someone to go in one direction, the human inclination is to choose the opposite. That's why when you seek therapists for some guidance, they usually don't tell you what to do. They help you find your own solutions. Therefore, if you change the wording to make it sound like the decision to take medication was made in collaboration with the patient, that they took part in choosing their treatment, then you will have better alliance and compliance.

When I give recommendations, I educate the patients first and give options with potential side effects, risks, and benefits. I say something like, "\_\_\_ is my best recommendation, but if you don't like\_\_\_\_ then \_\_\_\_\_ may be a better option for you because of\_\_\_\_." Or, "These two medications work about the same, but this one has \_\_\_\_ and that one has \_\_\_\_. Do you have a preference?" If you include your patients in the decision to choose that medication, then they are more likely to take it.

**Empathy goes a long way.** When I was a medical student in a mock interview with a patient, I asked all the right questions, got the correct diagnosis and plan, but I lost points on not having empathy. Back then, I thought, "Huh?! Empathy?!" Though I thought it was stupid to have "empathy" as part of the grading system, I did not disagree that my performance lacked empathy because I was more focused on what's wrong with the patient's body and how to fix it than the patient himself.

Now I believe in the power of empathy and how vital it is to connect with patients. I had a patient who had a rare skin disease and he itched so badly that he scratched off chunks of his skin flesh for some relief. You can't imagine how horrific he looks and the associated pain he feels from all the wounds. I placed my hand on my chest, looked at him with sadness, and said in a soft voice, "I am so sorry for all the suffering that you are going through. You must be in a lot of pain. I know it must have been hard for you to come to this appointment, so I will do my best to help you." His eyes glistened in tears. He was so grateful that I listened and cared, and that I took the time to validate his suffering. It takes five seconds to show empathy, but the effect on the patient will last for a long time.

All human beings want to be validated, to be seen, to be heard, to matter, and that's what we all should strive to do for our patients and for each other.

**Take the first few minutes to connect.** From the first moment that I see my patients, I put on a big smile because I want them to know that just seeing them makes me happy. Within the first few minutes of the appointment, I let them talk about whatever is on their mind, even if what they say has nothing to do with their medical needs. This tells them that I value what they want to bring up first because what they have to say is more important than my agenda for the appointment.

I had a patient who is into producing her own music. When she came into my office, she told me about how she asked a DJ to play her song at a party and everyone liked her music. She asked if I wanted to hear it and I said yes. She gave me a CD from her purse. We played it in my computer and she started to dance and I joined in, bopping my shoulders along with the beat. We listened to her music for couple of minutes. I praised her for how talented she was and how much I enjoyed the music. We then continued with the business of the appointment, and at the end, she thanked me for being "encouraging" and "wonderful" and listening to her music.

You may think, "What a waste of time. Those few minutes from every patient adds up at the end of the day." True, but I believe this saves a lot of time in the long run. When you show from the beginning that the patient is important to you and that you care about what's important to them, then they build trust in you and are more likely to agree with your recommended medication or treatment.

If you present your treatment plan without making the effort to connect, the trust isn't there. The patient might as well trust Google instead. He may argue against the recommended treatment, may question your motive, may not do exactly what you ask, all of which take a lot more time in the long run than the first few minutes of your first appointment.

## How to present to attendings

**Present only the salient points**. If your attending has any questions about your presentation, then you can present additional information then. I have presented many times to senior residents or attendings and I have been presented to many times by junior residents or interns. Having been on both sides, I get it.

When I used to present as an intern, I presented ALL the information that I gathered from the patient. I thought being thorough and detail-oriented were positive attributes but not from the attendings' perspective. I could see how quickly I was losing their attention in the middle of my presentation. They would look away, type on their laptops, or check their phones. Hello? I'm trying to tell you about our patient!

From the attending's perspective, less is better. When I was a senior resident listening to interns present, I was the same way—impatiently waiting for the bottom line. I wanted them to just get to the point and tell me what I NEED to know, not everything they know. You should have a good reason to present everything you present. If it's just an extra detail that has no effect on the diagnosis or plan, don't mention it.

If you do not know what the salient points are—what you should or should not present—then listen to the other interns and residents. Every rotation requires different relevant information that should be presented. If you do not have a chance to listen in, then read other residents' notes. Note what they add and omit, and use that as a guide. That should give you a good start until you figure out what is important and what is not.

## How to write notes

Documentation is a form of communication and a reflection of who you are and how you practice. Many people will read your notes and rely on you to communicate clearly.

**Look at previous notes.** Every rotation and site has a different type of note, just as mentioned previously regarding presentations. Some places provide their template and some just a piece of blank paper. No need to reinvent the wheel. Just look at how other doctors have written their notes, which hopefully are good notes, and write something similar.

**Write concisely with substance.** Forget what you learned in school about avoiding incomplete or run-on sentences. No one will care how you write;they'll only care about what you write. Keep your notes short and include only relevant information. For example, write, "Denies side effects," instead of, "Patient denies having any side effect to taking her medications." Two or three words can convey the same information as ten words. Writing concisely saves time for both the writer and the reader.

**What's a good note?** At a minimum, write what's going on (past history and diagnosis) and what's the plan. If your note is too long, people just skim and may miss the point you are trying to get across. If it's too short without any substance, then it's useless. Your colleagues and team members depend on your note to care for your patient, so make sure your note is concise with relevant information.

When I transitioned from second to third year of residency, I replaced another resident's position in a university clinic, so I had taken over all his patients. Every time I had a patient scheduled I read his previous notes to see what I could gather before seeing the patient for the first time. Because the previous resident's notes contained so much useful content, I probably gathered about 80% of all the information I needed from his notes and 20% from the patients. Even before I saw my patients I felt like I really knew them. I contacted this resident to say big, "thank you" for making the transition of care smooth for the patients and easy for me.

Writing good notes is also important because if there is a lawsuit involving your patient, your note will be read and scrutinized in detail. If you did something but did not write it in your note, by the time the lawsuit is filed and you are questioned, you may not remember if you actually did it or not. And in the eyes of the law, you did not do what you don't remember doing and what you did not document doing, and you may be liable for it.

**What's a bad note?** Sometimes I see notes like, "Doing well. Gave Invega." That's it. My thoughts on this is that this doctor literally saw the patient for a minute, didn't ask many questions, and just gave the monthly shot. Maybe he didn't bother to write anything more because he saw no need. Maybe he just doesn't care about his patient or his job. Writing four words in a progress note does not leave a good impression whether you are an attending or a resident.

When this doctor left his job and I took over his patients, I spent so much time trying to gather history on all his patients and figure out what's going on. It was a nightmare for me and for patients as well because most patients do not know their medical history. They say something like, "I used to take that small white pill," like I'm supposed to know what that is. They also say, "I tried some medications, but I don't remember what they are." What am I supposed to do? I have to start from scratch. The worst is when they say, "Isn't it in my record?" Because then, I have to apologize on behalf of their previous doctor.

## How to be a great doctor

Your patients do not care about all the details of the biological pathways, receptors, half-lives, 20-plus list of side effects, etc. They just want to know if they were heard and if you cared. You do that by being nice, treating them kindly and with respect.

**Show respect.** Part of showing respect is respecting your patients' time. When you are late to an arranged meeting time, it implies that your time is more important than that of the person who was waiting for you. Some doctors routinely see their patients 30-plus minutes after the appointment time. If you have been a patient yourself, you know how annoying that is and how that affects the rest of your day.

As a doctor, I consider myself to be "working for" my patients, so in essence, they are like my bosses. I treat them with respect and always make sure that I bring them into my office on time. And in rare occasions I am late, the first thing I say is an apology for being late.

You may say, "Well, if the patient before came in late, then I have to see the next patient late." This doesn't make sense. Why punish the patient who was on time for the sake of the patient who was late? When my patient is late, the appointment is shortened and I still finish on time. If my patient is really late, then I reschedule.

You may say the patient was a complicated case, or very sick, or needed interpreting service. Well then, you better work fast. No more excuses. Make it a MUST that you start and finish on time for your patient, and it will happen.

I have had so many patients thank me for taking them in on time and I had zero patients complain that the appointment was short because they came in late.

**It's not about you.** You will always have that patient who gets on your nerves, who's just plain old mean, who doesn't listen to your recommendations and still complains that you need to do something, who blames you for their bad health, who frequently doesn't show up for appointments, who calls you by your first name or Mr./Mrs. instead of doctor, or who says how he knows more than you because he googled it.

It is so easy to lose your temper, express your annoyance, or even show some passive aggression, but don't do it. No matter what your patient says or does, the appointment is all about your patient, not you.

Even if your patient asks, "How are you, doctor?" Besides saying "good" or "fine," you shouldn't add anything more. It's not your place to say how your day has been, how you were annoyed by the traffic in the morning, or how your arthritis is acting up. It's human nature to want to talk about yourself, but as a doctor, you have to resist this urge and make the conversation only about the patient.

**Be quick to apologize and quick to agree.** When there is fire, extinguish it as quickly as possible. Some patients come to me wearing boxing gloves, figuratively, and ready to fight. I have a patient who has history of aggression and violence. When we first met, he walked into my office with wide strides and stiffened angry face. I tried asking some common gentle questions and he was quick to respond with, "Who the f--- do you think you are? You don't know me! You don't know what I've been through! You f---ing shrink!"

I responded, "I'm so sorry. I didn't mean to upset you. You're right. I don't know you, but I would like to get to know you more so I can find ways to help you. Is that okay?" My response took him off guard. He probably imagined us in a boxing ring, he gave his best shot, and he was ready to get punched back. But I quickly took off my gloves and kneeled in defeat, figuratively, of course. As quickly as he was fired up to yell at me, after my quick, sincere apology, he calmed down right away.

Needless to say, this patient now comes to see me with big smiles, excitedly tells me about his latest project he's been working on. I reflect the excitement and tell him what a great job he's doing and compliment how creative he is.

**Keep learning.** Medical knowledge changes all the time, so you have an important duty to keep your knowledge current.

As a resident, it's important to know at least the basics. I often read medical textbooks and journals. I also tried to learn as much as I could from my supervisors and attendings.

After residency, I learn and get new updates mainly from email listserv, online, and collaboration with other doctors. Since I work for two counties, the medical directors often email me if there is a new FDA warning or other important matters. Other doctors I work with share relevant information as well. I also present complicated cases to my fellow doctors, and I'm often part of the discussion of their difficult cases.

**Take advantage of your supervision.** As a resident, you have supervisors and attendings easily available to you. Take full advantage of these free luxuries. I used to just "show up" to my supervisions because I was required to, but soon, I realized how much I was learning and how valuable these times were.

The knowledge I gained from my supervisor's experience was not accessible by books or Google. So before every supervision hour, I prepared questions or cases, and I wrote notes during supervision as well. Afterwards, I transferred my notes to a Word document and reviewed them periodically to solidify the knowledge. I wish I had known how precious these times were earlier in my residency training, so I could have gained and retained more knowledge.

**Practice what you preach.** You are in the business of providing service to promote health, not just treating illness. If you don't practice healthy living yourself, how can you convince your patients to do the same? You may say, "But that patient is over 300 lbs with high cholesterol, diabetes, and hypertension. He's the one who really needs to lose weight. I'm just big boned." Being healthy is for everyone, fat or skinny, including doctors, not just patients.

After residency, I put more focus on my own health because I felt like a hypocrite telling my patients to get healthier when I was unhealthy and overweight. I made dietary, fitness, and lifestyle changes to become healthy, some of which I discussed in a previous chapter. Now when I tell my patients how to lose weight and keep themselves healthy, I say it with enthusiasm and passion. I share recipes and pictures of the food I prepare. I share some exercise routines that I do. I tell them, "This is how I did it. So, you can do it, too." Then, one by one, patients come to me and tell me how they have been taking their steps to be healthy like drinking healthy smoothies, adding more vegetables to their meals, walking more, and it feels so rewarding to see such change in them.

# HOW TO Do the Rest

Studying for board exam, finding a job, and trying to find ways to pay your debt are all important part of your residency. Residents often worry about the HOW. How do you study for board exam? How am I supposed to find a job? How do I pay for my debt? All these HOW questions are addressed in this chapter.

**How to study for board exam**

Most residents take about a week off of work to study for the board exam. If you have always done well on standardized exams like Steps 1, 2, and 3, then, you'll probably do fine studying for a week. I, on the other hand, have never been a stellar test taker. I took PRITE exams, which are two half-day practice exams with questions that are similar to the board exams. All psychiatry residents take this exam once a year starting the second year and you are scored and ranked along with your classmates. As a second year resident, I took the test the morning after a call night and I was too tired to focus on the test. So, to no surprise, I did poorly and ranked sixth out of six residents in my class. As a third year resident, I no long had the excuse of being post-call and I figured I could only go up from the last place. I was wrong. I remained at the last place. For my fourth year, I studied hard for a month and was convinced that if I studied hard I would not be ranked last in my class. The scores came in. I scored the best compared to my previous scores, but I was still in sixth place. So I knew I needed help to study for my boards, and a week of studying on my own was not going to cut it.

**Should I take the board exam?** Before you decide to study for a board exam, you may wonder if you even need to take the exam. The answer is no, you do not have to, but you should.

First, there is some recognition given to doctors if "board certified" is placed before their names. It may not be a big deal to doctors but patients' opinions are different – to them board certification means that you are more knowledgeable, reliable, and accomplished. If you listen to the radio or television about some advertisement of treatment or procedure, listen for how they introduce the doctor. You often hear, "Dr. So-and-so is board certified…"

Another reason to be board certified is that most employers want their doctors to be board certified, so they usually offer monetary incentives to obtain it. For example, my hourly salary increased $10 per hour after I obtain my board certification. My friend receives an additional $5000 per year because she is board certified.

**What tools to use to study for the board exam?** Ask around. There are many options, so you should think about which option would work for you. One of my supervisors recommended BeattheBoards.com, which is an online site that provides study guides with many lectures, practice questions, and outlines to help you pass the exam. My biggest reservation was the cost, which was about a thousand dollars. But I reasoned that the money was worth spending because when I graduate I would be making about $1000 in less than a day's work. Additionally, if you do not pass after using this program, the company offers a full refund plus additional 10% back, and you have continuing access until you pass. You can also get a referral discount of $52 by mentioning the person who referred you, and you are welcome to mention my name.

I signed up for BeattheBoards.com about five months before my board exam and studied almost every night for about 30 to 45 minutes while I was putting my kids to sleep. I wish I had used the program earlier since it offers a one-year subscription and because I applied a lot of what I learned into my clinical practice. By the time I took the exam, I felt confident and finished over an hour before the finish time.

## How to get a job

The hardest or the easiest part of finding a job is knowing what you want. Do you want to stay in the area or move to your home town? Do you want to work in a hospital setting or in outpatient only? Do you want to work part-time or full-time? Once you decide what kind of work you want, the rest is easy.

**Ask for an interview.** When you look for a job as a doctor, you can go straight to the site where you want to work and ask for an interview, in case they will hire in the near future. You can get a better feel for how your work life will be like if you are actually at the work site meeting the people you'll be working with. I asked for interviews from my two current employers without even knowing if they had any job opening.

**Ask around and use your connections.** Some residents get jobs from asking around through word-of-mouth.

When I was considering going into private practice, one of my supervisors introduced me to a colleague that she knew long time ago in the area where I wanted to practice. I contacted him, mentioning my supervisor's name and he invited me to his home, talked to me for couple of hours, showed me his private practice office, and offered me opportunity to work in his office building. Now that's the power of using your connections!

There was another doctor with whom I wanted to work, but I didn't know anyone who knew him. So, I called his phone number from his website and left a message. His secretary called me back few days later and told me that I needed to read his book first before I could talk to him. My guess is that if I had named someone that he knew, saying, "Dr. So-and-so told me to talk to you," he would not have required that I read his book.

**Start the process EARLY in the beginning of your last year of residency.** Finding a job was relatively easy for me because I knew exactly what I wanted. I had to find an outpatient job in Northern Virginia, which limited my choices. I had considered and interviewed for jobs with call duty, but later decided I did not want any calls in my schedule. Based on these criteria, the only option was to work for the county. I contacted the medical directors of two counties near where I will live after residency and asked for an interview early in the last year of my residency. Through the rest of that year, I kept in touch, just to let them know, "Hey, I'm still interested in working there."

The reason why you should apply early is because it takes time to get hired. There is a lot of paperwork and there are many delays for various reasons. The earlier you know where you want to work, the better chance you have to start working immediately after residency.

Another reason to start the process early is so the employers will think of you when a position opens up. I expressed strong interest in one site, and reminded the director throughout the year that I was still interested in that site. Two months before my residency graduation, a doctor at that site decided to quit to move out of state, and guess who was in the director's mind to replace her? Me!

## How to determine what a job entails

In order to know about the job that you are considering, it is critical to ask the following questions.

**How is the call schedule?** Being on call during residency is very different from being on call after residency. It's not enough to ask how many calls you would have in a month or a year. Ask about what work is entailed during a call.

A call during weekend can mean you come to work and see ALL the patients in the hospital unit and write ALL the notes on those patients, which means all day of a lot of work. A call can also mean coming to work to only see new patients or not coming to work and instead get called on the phone for orders. One job I considered had two call schedules per month, one weekend and one weekday. A call for this job meant phone calls only, but it also meant frequently taking calls throughout the night and still having a full work schedule the following day. At another job, if you're on call during a weekend, you are off on Monday and Tuesday.

There are a lot of variations of what a "call" is, so ask for details. I had a friend who was working in his "ideal" job. However, he didn't like being on call every third weekend, so he quit. After two years, his job position was still not filled.

**How is work life?** Ask to speak to the doctors already working at the job you want to consider. Besides listening for the answers to your questions, notice how they respond. Do they really seem as though they like their job? Are they saying more about their job besides just answering your questions? Listen carefully for what is said and not said.

I spoke to one doctor about a potential job and though he was answering my questions, his answers were vague and brief. He did not sound enthusiastic about his work. Even when I asked if there was anything else I should know, he answered, "No." Something just didn't feel right in my gut.

When I was interviewing for another job, the first thing that came out of the medical director's mouth was about billing, how I had to bill certain number of hours and those who didn't were let go in the past. I think I would have been fine with billing requirement since I pride myself in working efficiently, but I certainly didn't want the pressure on my shoulders that if I didn't meet the quota then I would be fired. That is not the kind of work environment I wanted.

When I interviewed for my current job, one doctor said, "You'll love this job. This is like a mom's job. The hours are flexible. No calls. You have a lot of freedom." I didn't even ask anything. She was selling the position on her own. She had been working in that job for about six years and she loves it. This spoke volumes to me.

**What do you like or dislike about your job?** Chances are what your potential coworkers like or dislike about their jobs will be the same things that you would like or dislike.

**How long have you and the other doctors worked here?** This question is important to know because if doctors come and go like a revolving door, that means something about the work is not fitting for many doctors.

When I was interviewing, there was one job site where the majority of doctors worked only for a year or two. I didn't know why, but I didn't feel that I had to. Something about the job was pushing doctors out the door, and I did not want to be one of them.

At my current two jobs, most doctors I work with have been working there for many years. This says a lot about job satisfaction. Something must be right with the job that everyone who works there STAYS, and that matters.

**How many minutes do you get to see a patient for new intake and for follow up? How many patients do you see per day?** Healthcare has unfortunately become more about business and profitability than providing quality care. The less time you have to see a patient, more often you have to rush, cut corners, and may even miss important history or symptoms. Some places expect you to see over 30 patients a day, some far fewer. As a county psychiatrist, I get about 30 mins to see follow-up patients, which includes 20 minutes of face time and 10 minutes of note writing. A friend of mine who works for a private group practice in the same field told me she has 20 minutes per patient, which includes writing notes. However, she does get some administrative time in the day.

**Are the hours flexible?** Some doctors prefer to work four days of ten hours per day, some prefer to have two half-days in the week, and some want every other Friday off. I prefer a schedule that allows me to drop off and pick up my kids from school. Having flexible work hours that meet your life needs is sometimes the most important reason to take or not take the job.

I interviewed at a job site where they ask the doctor to work from 12 pm to 8 pm with no flexibility of hours. Even if the pay and everything else were perfect, I couldn't even consider this job because I would not be able to pick up my kids from school and would be missing dinner with my family.

**How many vacation and sick days do you get per year?** In many places, the more years you work, the more vacation days you get. During the first year, you may get three weeks of vacation, but by the time you have worked at that location for 10 years, you may get six weeks off per year. One of my friends has three months of vacation per year! If you are a contractor, then you do not get paid vacation days, but you have the freedom to take as many vacation days as you want.

## How to determine where you want to work

The road commonly traveled by residents is working at a lucrative job with lots of benefits. This looks good on the paper, but they often must see many patients in a short amount of time with frequent call schedule and limited administrative support. If you would rather be busy and earn a lot of money with great perks, then this is a great option for you.

One of my colleagues told me about her first job after residency. The salary was very high, lots of benefits, and appeared pretty good on the surface. Once she started working, she was overwhelmed with the amount of work she had to do during the day with minimal support. She also had call scheduled every four days. She said she worked longer hours than when she was a resident, and that says a lot! Her contract was initially written for two years, which in itself should be suspicious, but at the advice of her lawyer, she asked for a one-year contract. She said she was so glad that she did because she quit as soon as her contract was over. Now she has a job that pays less but has a reasonable patient load, no calls, and where she sees herself eventually retiring.

**Private practice** is a popular option, as you can potentially make a lot of money and be your own boss—no one is telling you what to do. However, you also have a lot of expense to run the practice. Also there is a lot more that you have to do besides just seeing patients, including managing the business of private practice, marketing yourself, and doing a lot of administrative work.

For example, a private practice psychiatrist in or near D.C., who does not take insurance, can easily make $300,000 to $400,000 per year. However, you have to subtract all the costs related to having private practice, which can vary, from $15,000 to $50,000 per year. A full time employed psychiatrist makes about $160,000 to $200,000 per year.

Almost everyone I talked to who works in a private practice really likes working in that setting. Surprisingly, the most common, consistent complaint was loneliness.

**Locum Tenem** is another good option, which also pays very well, and is ideal for those who like traveling and want to see different parts of US. Locums usually work with a company that facilitates all of the paperwork and logistics. They tend to work about three months at a time, but sometimes they extend their contracts or decide to become employees afterwards. You do have to get licensed in every state in which you work, and some locum companies will pay for the licensing cost.

After a year of working in a hospital setting, one of my friends decided to work locum and she said that one site was paying her

$150 per hour plus benefits and an apartment. She was single, adventurous, and excited to travel. This kind of work fits her life and her personality.

**County/Community doctor** is another option and the work experience is different, depending on where you are.

One of the benefits of being a county/community doctor is that you get administrative support. In one of the counties I work for, I have my own dedicated nurse who takes care of all the correspondence, paperwork, and administrative work.

The challenge of working for the county or in an underserved area is that there is more demand (patients) than supply (doctors) with limited budget and available appointment times. Sometimes my schedule is booked two months out, which means that if one of my patients has to see me for an urgent matter, he will have to wait for someone in my schedule to cancel or go see another doctor at an urgent care.

Working for the county was my obvious choice because the county doctors where I work do not take any calls, which was important to me. A permanent employee position with benefits was not available, so I took a contract position with no benefits (no health insurance, no paid vacation, no paid holidays). It has a relatively low salary and is part-time (28 hours a week). Many residents would not even consider this option, but I felt this was the road meant for me.

Because I work part-time, the quality of my life is so much better! Not only do I get to spend more time with my family, but I get to pursue other interests like reading books, cooking healthy meals, Zumba dancing, and writing this book.

In summary, since you do have a lot of choices, think about what aspect of work life is most important to you. Some may choose the high paying job to make a lot of money and may even thrive in the high intensity, high volume patient load. Some may be sick and tired of having bosses and want the freedom to do whatever they want, so private practice may be a good option for them. Some may want to see different parts of the country and prefer to live like a nomad, so locum may be a good fit. If you are a parent and your spouse has a job with benefits, then a part-time contract position may be more appealing option for you.

## How to pay off your debt

The average medical student graduates with about $150,000 to $200,000 in debt. That is the average, but the range is wide. Some of my friends in medical school had rich parents who paid for all their tuition and living costs. They graduated with zero debt. And then there are those who accrued debt starting from undergraduate to graduate school and even more for medical school, all totaling $400,000 to $700,000 or more.

Nobody likes to talk about debt during medical school or residency. It is often swept under the rug until the last year when you have to face the growing, monstrous debt. While you were not paying your debt, it was just growing from accrued interest.

What do residents do? Some still spend money during residency as though they have unlimited income—going to expensive dinners, buying new clothes, going to extravagant vacations, renting luxury apartments, etc. They often say, "Who cares? I'm already $300,000 in debt, what's another $50." It is like a 400 pound obese person saying, "What's another ice cream? I'm already fat."

If you consider the total amount of debt, it can be overwhelming. Unless you are born to rich parents, married to a rich spouse, or win the lottery, you are stuck with the mountain of debt and the best way to pay it off is to just chip it away little at a time, as fast and as much as you can. However, there are other options.

One of my friends' job has a loan forgiveness program, where she's given a total of $120,000 if she works in that job for five years. Sounds great, huh? However, she also mentioned that on many days she sees around 13 patients and sometimes as many as five to seven new intakes a day. To put this in perspective, in any given full day of work, I see about eight to ten patients with one new intake.

I knew a child psychiatrist who was earning well over $200,000 in an underserved area and who was taking advantage of a loan forgiveness program. He was seeing over 20 patients per day with no administrative time, so he stayed late every day to finish all his notes.

What I realized is that loan forgiveness programs sound great, but free money is not really free. You typically work long hours and see more patients in jobs that offer such incentive. When it looks too good to be true, be suspicious and ask yourself, "What's the catch?" Maybe it's that you get burned out or that you barely get to spend time with your family during weekdays.

Another loan forgiveness option is a 10-year loan repayment/forgiveness program. In this program, after paying your loan and working in nonprofit or public jobs for 10 years, the remainder of your debt is forgiven by the government. For more information, go to https://studentaid.ed.gov/sa/repay-loans/forgiveness-cancellation/public-service. I considered this option and asked my husband for his thoughts. He wanted me to have the freedom to work wherever I want and however long I want, so he did not like this option. Freedom is priceless. There is a difference in your spirit when you are working at a job because you have to verses working at a job because you want to.

I graduated from medical school with $200,000 in debt, which would have been a lot more if I had been on my own. Since my husband was working while I was going to medical school, he paid for all of our living expenses during that time. Even during residency we paid off our debt as much as we could. Every extra dollar that wasn't used up at the end of the month went to paying off the debt.

I set a goal to pay off my debt within two years after graduating from medical school, and two years later, we were debt free. We were able to pay it off because this was a goal that I told myself I MUST do, so all my daily decisions, conscious and subconscious, were aligned with this goal, just like my prior goal to have a wonderful residency experience.

Only through mindfully making multiple small decisions in the day to spend less or not at all were we able to pay off our $200,000 debt in two years. We continued to live in small places and live minimally. Every time I thought of buying something I asked myself, "Do I need this or want this?" I made frugal choices, buying used furniture from Craigslist or getting it free from family members. I tried to cook food to feed the family of four for less than $10 a meal. We rarely went out to eat and when we did, we went to less expensive restaurants. Even looking at a menu, I usually ordered cheaper options or eat an appetizer as a meal. When I did get my food, I tried to save half to eat for lunch the following day. Paying off $200,000 in two years is the result of all these small decisions.

When I was a resident, I noticed a resident friend had a nice outfit, so I complimented her. She told me how she signed up for this company that sends her a complete outfit once a month. I also happened to know that she gets her eyebrows professionally plucked and takes aerobics classes. She also told me she had over $100,000 in student debt, and she was curious to know how I paid of my $200,000 debt in two years during residency.

The reality is that $100,000 of debt would bother me enough to pluck my own eyebrows, but it doesn't bother my friend. She would rather have a little luxury in her life now and pay off her the debt later. It's a matter of personal preference. However, if you WANT to get rid of your debt in a specified timeframe and you DECIDE that you HAVE to do it, then the thought of buying new outfit every month, buying a new car instead of pre-owned, or any kind of purchase that you want instead of need does not even enter into your mind because these things pull you further from your desired goal. So, paying off your debt quickly starts with your desire and your decision to make it happen.

# Final Thoughts

For many years, you have wanted to be a doctor. Now you are at the final stretch to being on your own. After you graduate from residency, what's next? Is it just being a doctor, working eight to five? Is it to make an income to finally purchase a home, pay the bills, save for retirement, like what everyone else does? I challenge you to see the road less traveled and ask, "What am I passionate about?"

After I achieved my goal of becoming a doctor and finishing residency, I decided to dream bigger dreams and to bring glory to God. Writing this book is my first project that I feel passionate about. When I was teaching in the Teaching Committee during residency, I felt like I had so much to teach and share, but not enough time or audience for doing so. Mentoring and giving advice to a handful of residents were great, but I always felt hungry to help more residents. So, I decided to write this book to reach bigger audience of all residents, and even medical students, so they too can learn to be efficient, productive, have better quality of life, and be happy.

What's in your heart?

# Thank you

Thank you so much for reading this book. If you have learned and benefited from this book, please give me an honest review so others may benefit as well. And, please share this book with your residency or medical school class, so they can also achieve a greater quality of residency life. I would really appreciate it.

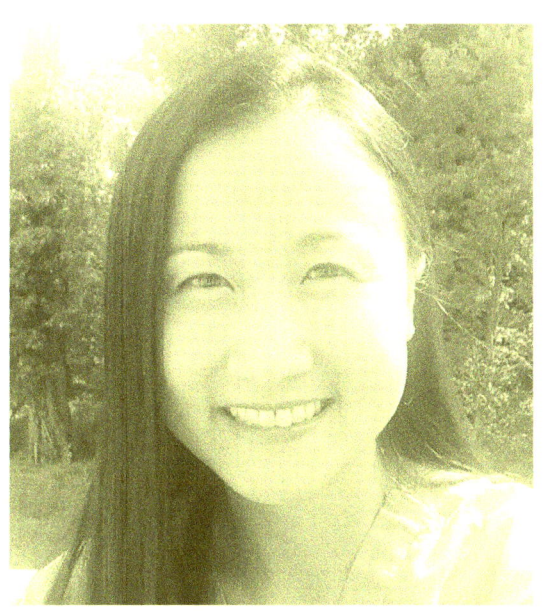

## About the author

Dr. Jenny Yi is a board certified psychiatrist in Northern Virginia. She received a Bachelor's degree from University of Virginia in 2000. She then attended Gallaudet University with an externship at the Mayo Clinic, and received her Doctorate of Audiology in 2004. After working as an audiologist at University of California, San Francisco, she decided to change her career and entered George Washington University Medical School in 2005. She took a year off during medical school to take care of her first child. She entered George Washington University Psychiatry Residency Program in 2010, and again took another year off to care for her second child. She graduated from residency in 2015, and is living happily with her two children and her loving husband. This is Dr. Yi's first book, but God willing, there will be many more to come.

www.ingramcontent.com/pod-product-compliance
Lightning Source LLC
Chambersburg PA
CBHW060355190526
45169CB00002B/602